Department of Neurosurgery,
University of GIESSEN, F. R. Germany
(Director: Prof. Dr. Dr. h. c. H. W. Pia)

EXPERIMENTAL NEUROSURGERY

H. W. Pia and R. Schönmayr
with drawings by L. Hettler (Lucky)

Walter de Gruyter · Berlin · New York 1981

This book can be received through an advanced payment of 14 German marks paid to Walter de Gruyter & Co., Genthiner Str. 13, D-1000 Berlin 30.

Introduction

This book with exercises in microneurosurgery is based on 13 years of experience in experimental and clinical microsurgery. It was originally prepared in 1979 as a set of instructions for microsurgery courses in Bombay, Calcutta and New Delhi and met with great demand. Also the trainees in our own laboratory found it very helpful in their daily practice.

This booklet is addressed to the young neurosurgeons and to all surgeons who begin their training in microsurgery. A simple description of the technique of suturing small vessels and nerves should help them to learn the microsurgical technique and to practice it in such a way as to acquire the necessary dexterity before attempting the microsurgical technique in human.

We would like to thank the de Gruyter Verlag - Berlin - New York for publishing this booklet and for keeping its price as low as possible.

Giessen, June 1981

H. W. Pia and
R. Schönmayr

TABLE OF CONTENTS

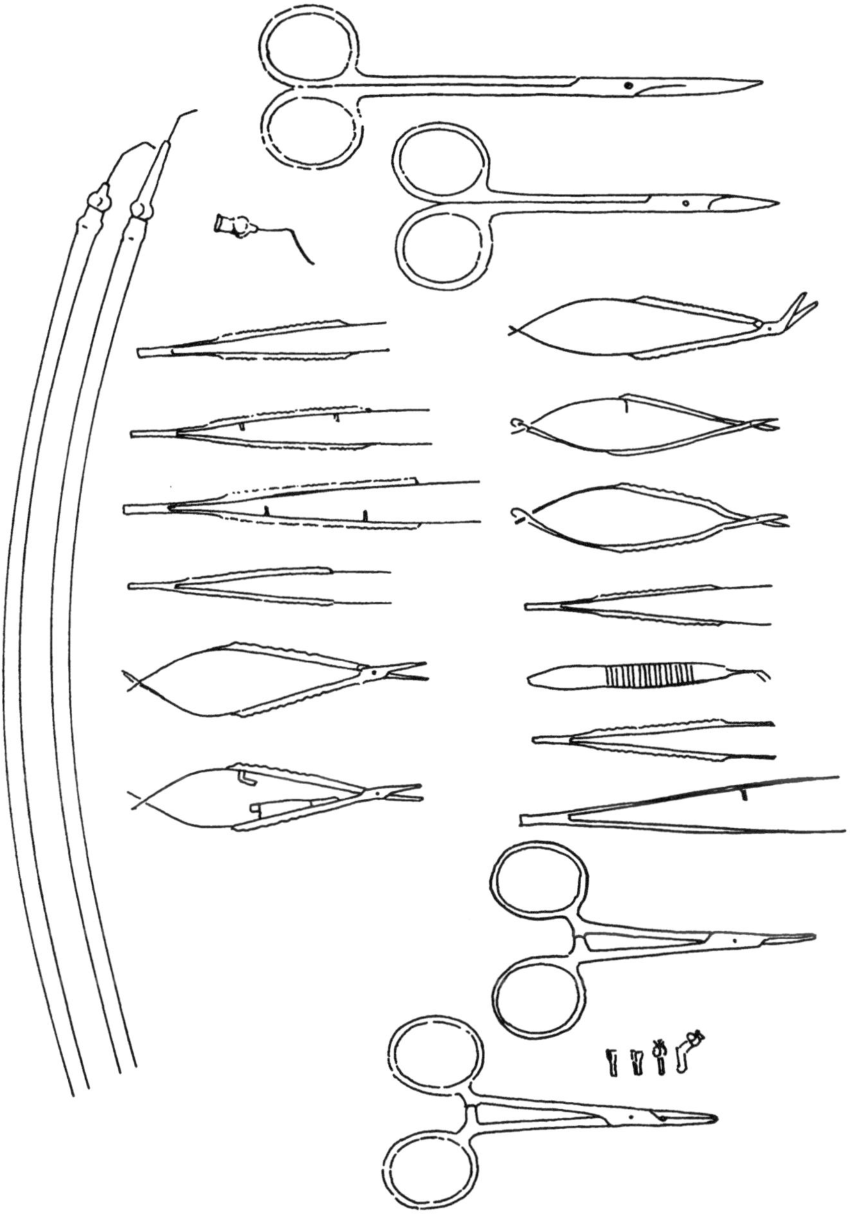

Instruments :

<u>Macro</u> (but small) :
Scalpel
Scissors
Forceps
"Retractors" :

you bend a canula to a hook and fix it with tape :

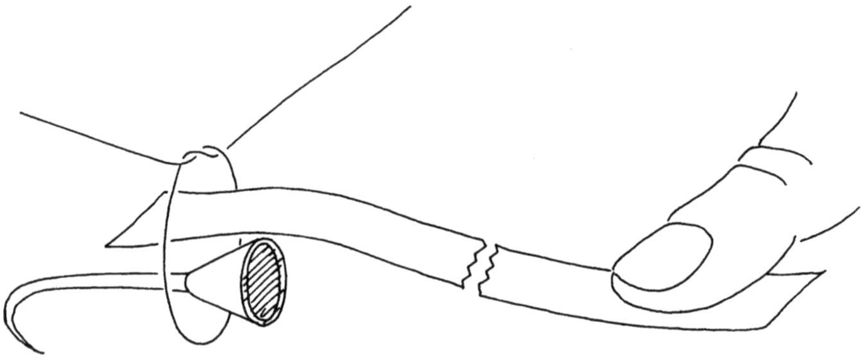

Sodium - Chloride Solution in a 5 cc syringe to keep wet the exposed tissue (the heat of the microscope - lamp would dry it within minutes).

<u>Important :</u> A piece of rubber 1 X 0,5 cm to put under the vessels.

Micro

Forceps (2)
Scissors
Tying-forceps
Needle-holder
Suture material (atraumatic) (10-0)

To flush the vessels take a 2 cc syringe and attach a 1 mm Ø baby vein-catheter:

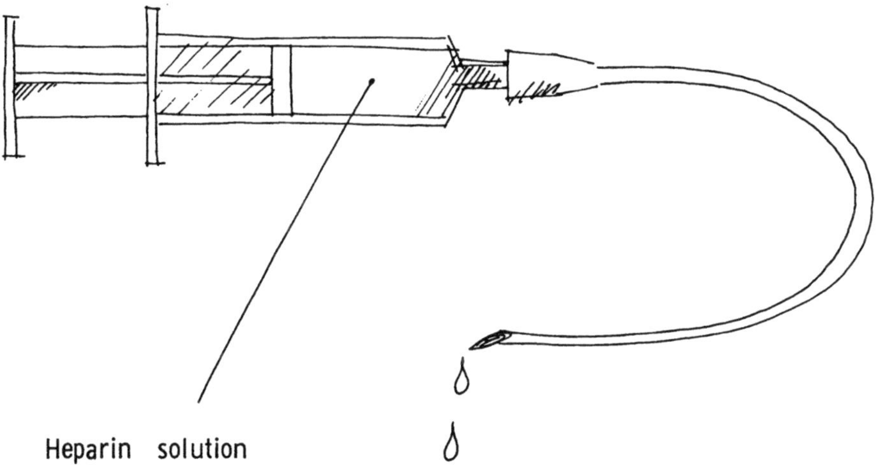

if possible:
bipolar coagulation
Clips

For Guineapig (Wt. 5oo g)
8 mg/cc Pentothal Sodium
intraper. - 1 Shot (Wait for
1o min.)

Rat

Anesthesia: intraperitoneal 1-2 cc

Thalamonal^{R} =
Droperidol (2.5 - 5 mg) + Fentanyl (o.o5 - o.1 mg)

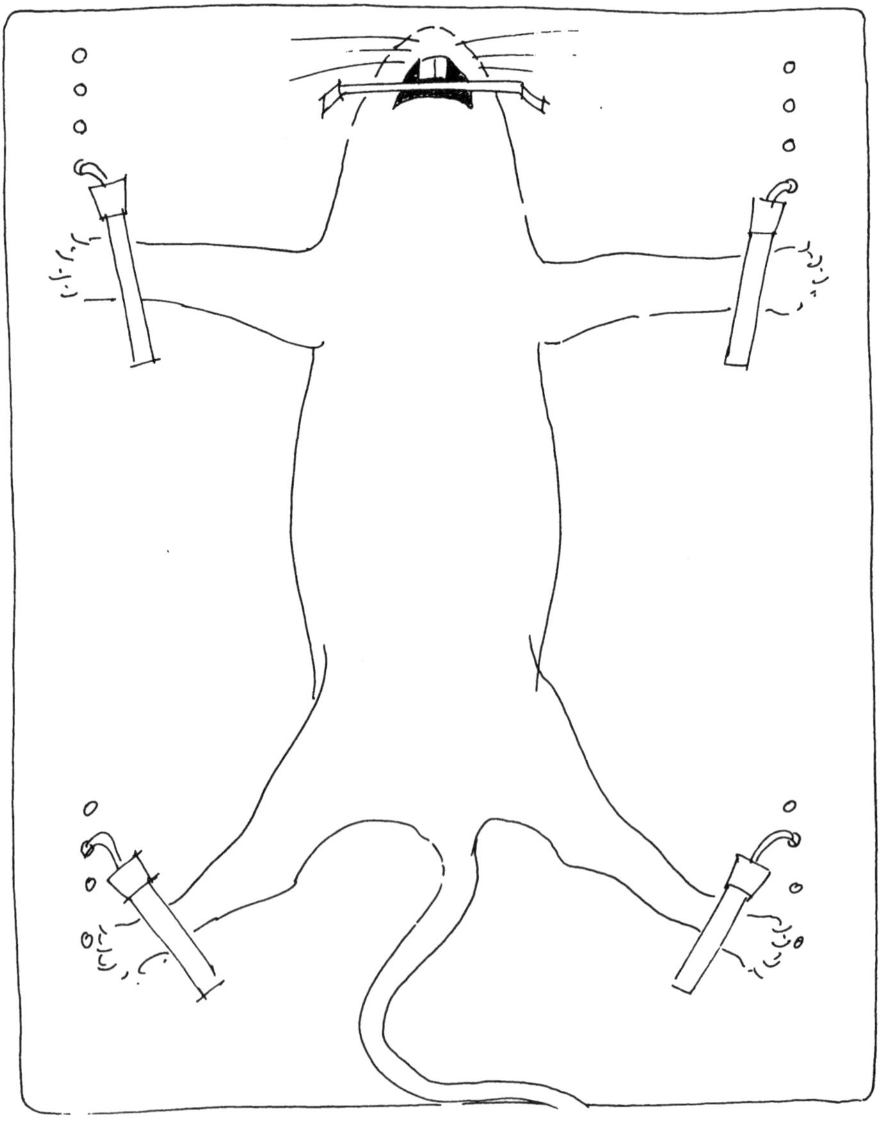

Skin incision

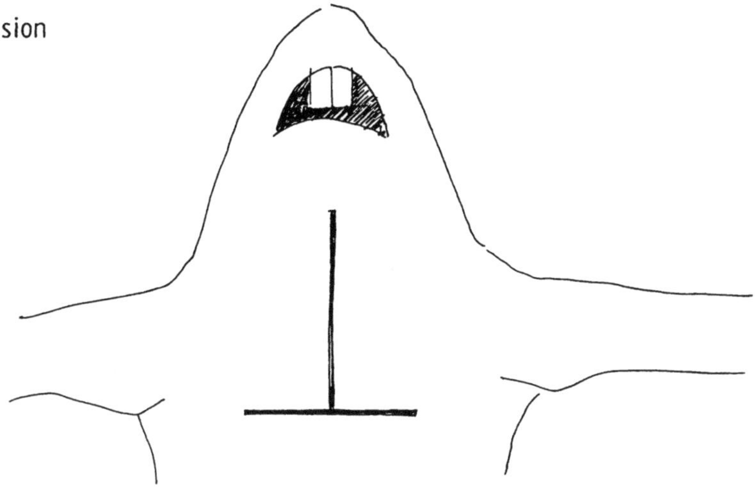

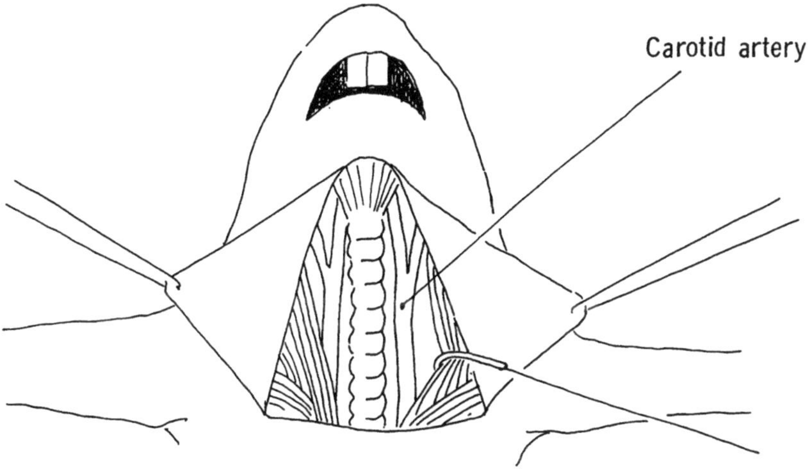

Important ! Keep the tissue wet by frequent application of saline-solution !

1) Temporary occlusion with clips:

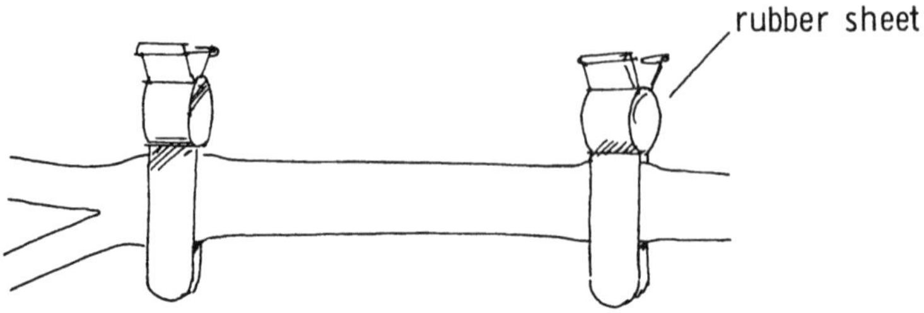

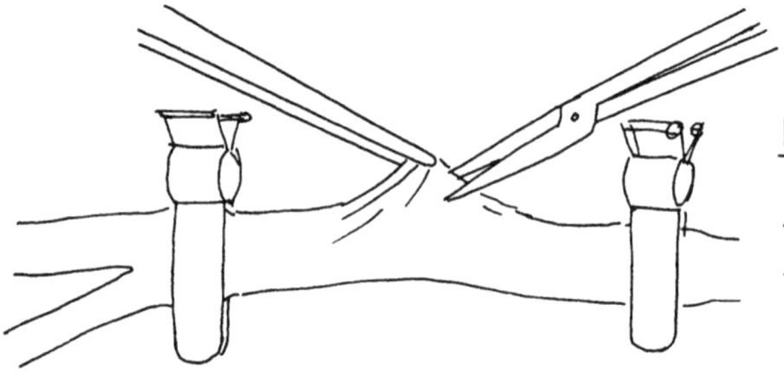

Important

Remove the highly thrombogenic adventitial tissue

Use sharp dissection without damaging the media

2) Longitudinal suture :

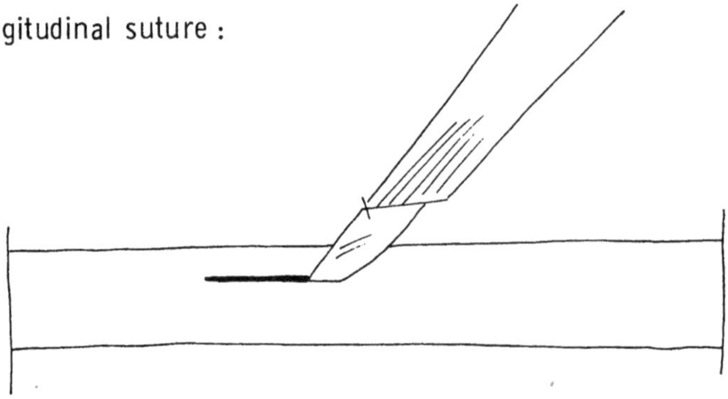

Longitudinal incision (razor blade)

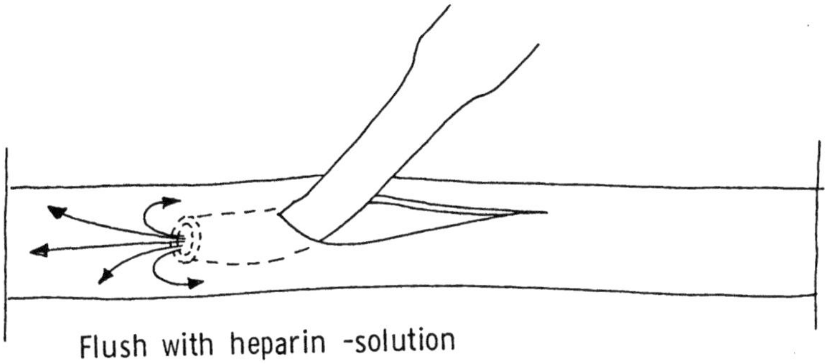

Flush with heparin -solution

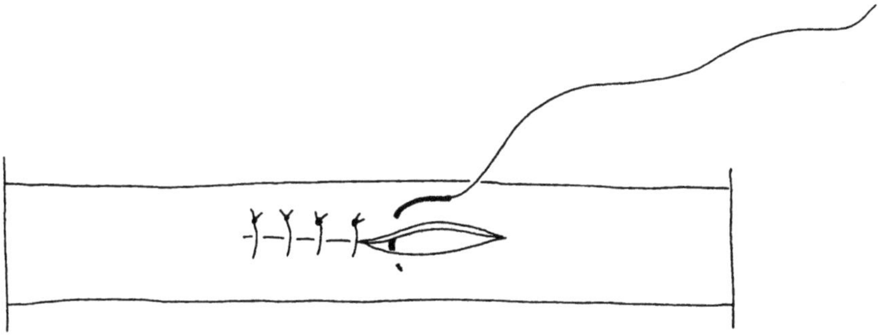

A) Single stitches:
Important: make sure to perforate all layers of the vascular wall. Try to set the stitches as close to the edge of the incision as possible, to avoid stenosis.

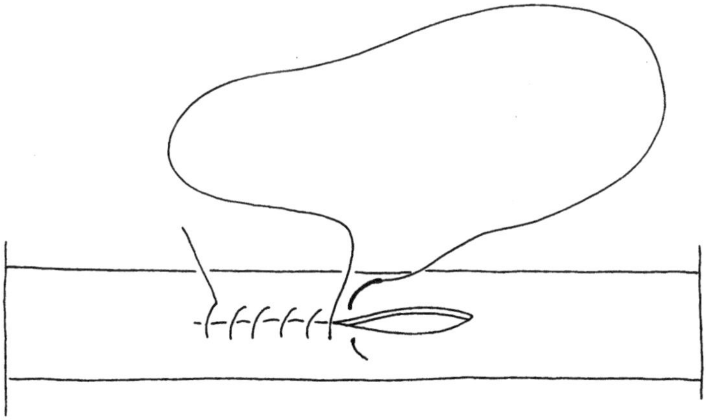

B) Continuous suture

Variation

Longitudinal suture over a tube:

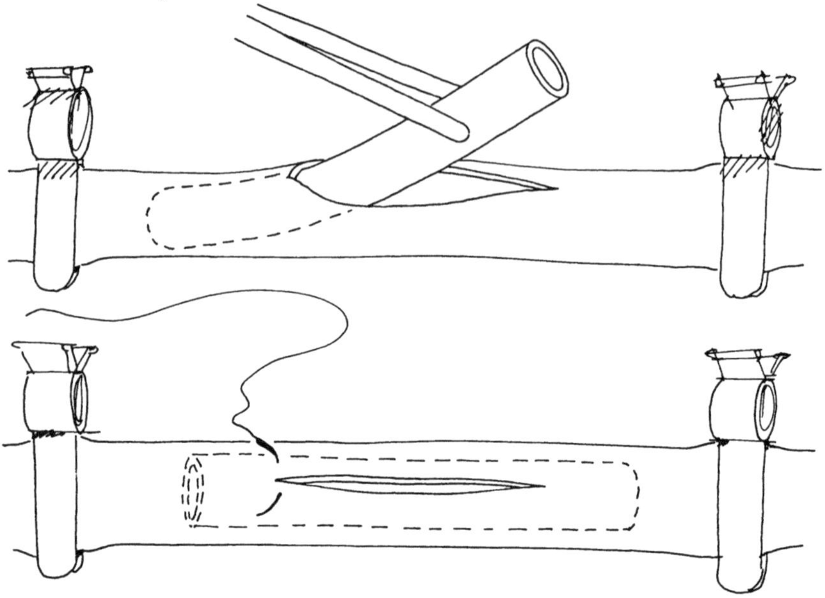

If you wish, you may remove the clips after slight fixation of the tube:

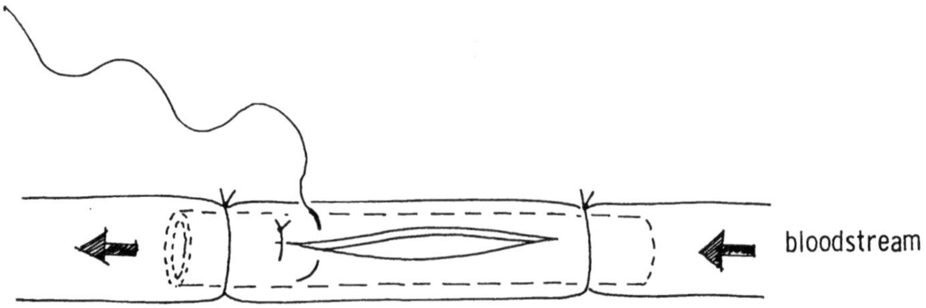

In this case flush tube before with heparin solution !

Remove the tube after clipping the vessel again.
Remove it before the last two stitches.

Important: flush out all blood with heparin solution before setting and tying the last two stitches.

3) End to End Anastomosis

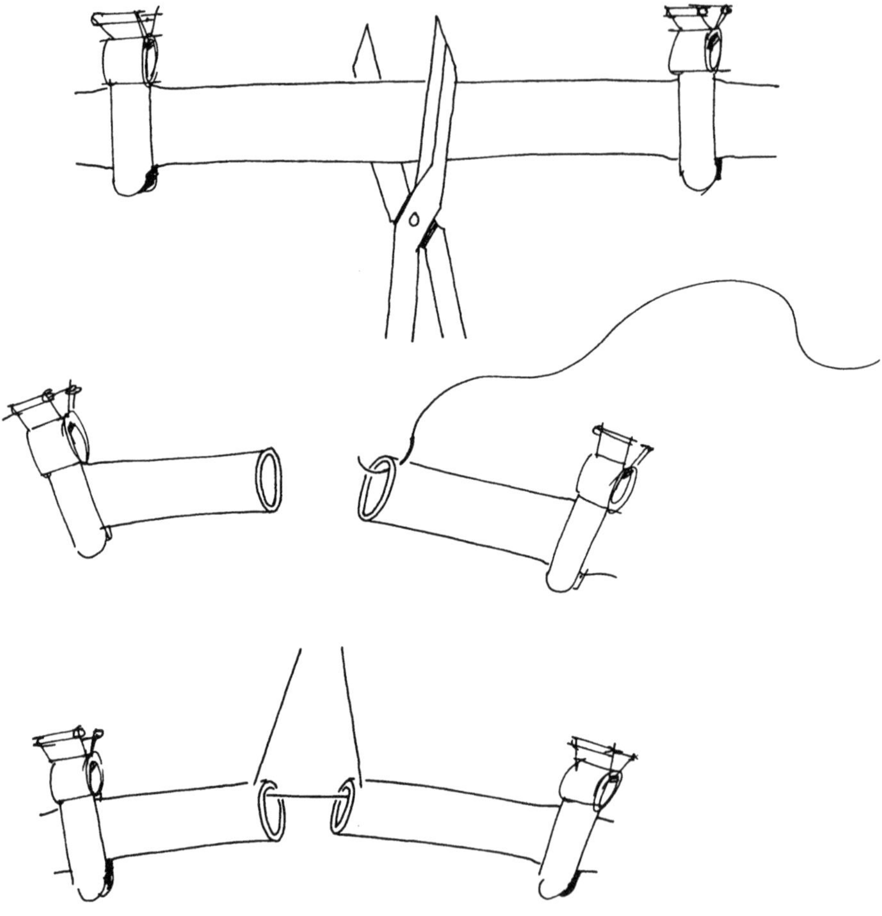

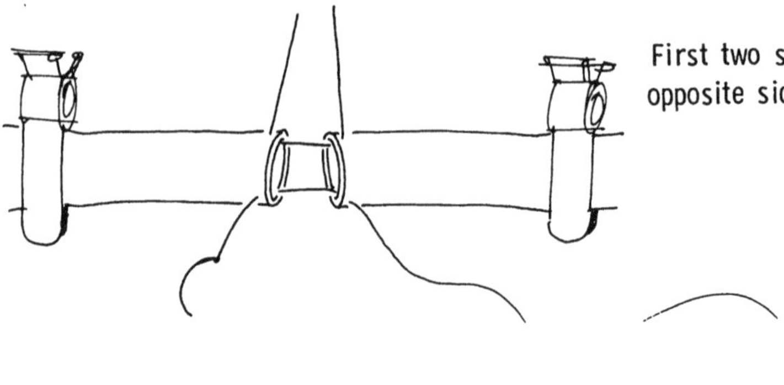

First two sutures on opposite sides

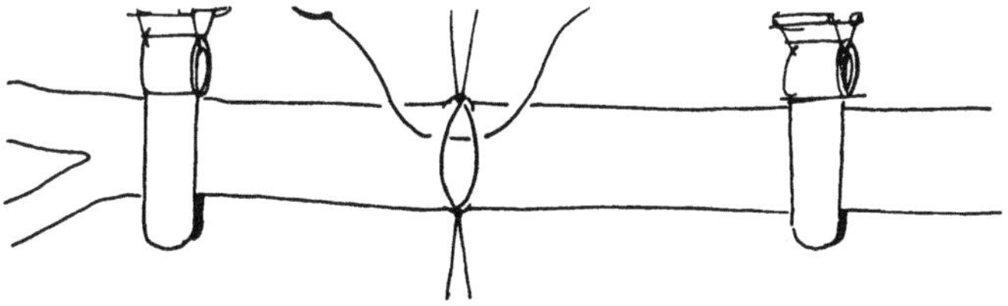

Better: after tying the initial fixation stitches leave the thread long in order to facilitate later rotation of the vessel.

After the suture of the anterior wall

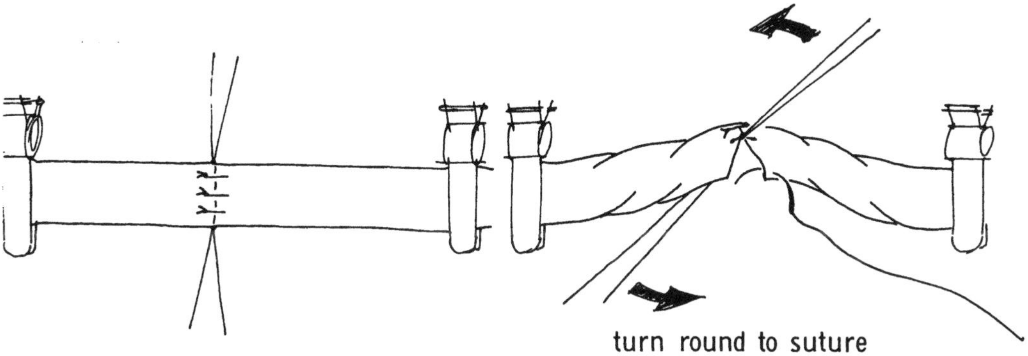

turn round to suture the opposite side.

Variation:
End to End suture over a tube:

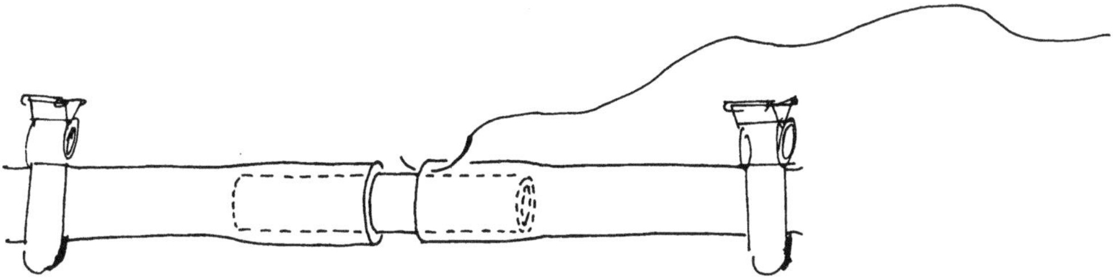

Do not forget to remove the tube before setting the last two stitches.
No matter if you use a tube or not, flush the clipped vessel with heparin solution before setting and tying the last two stitches!

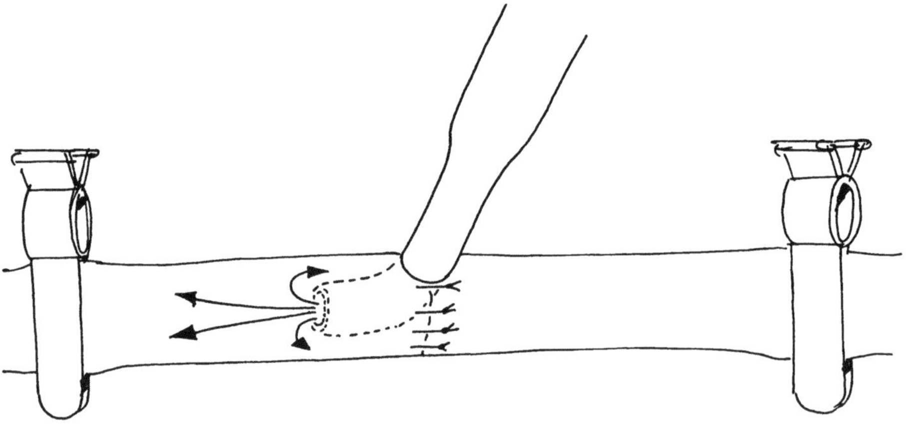

4) <u>Patch :</u>

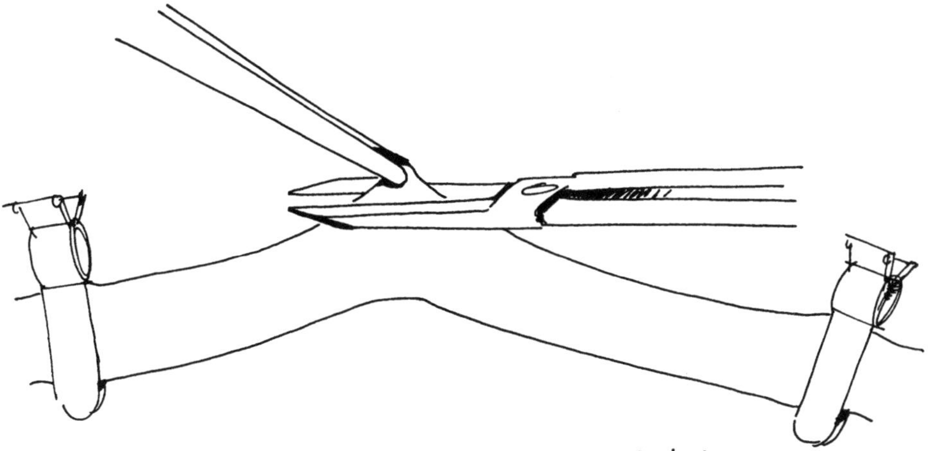

Excision of the arterial wall.

Preparation of a fitting venous (or arterial) patch:

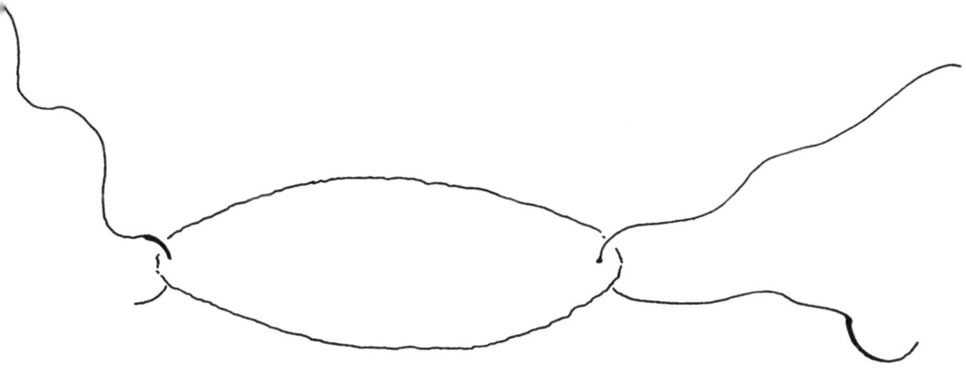

Patch (Vein, Artery)

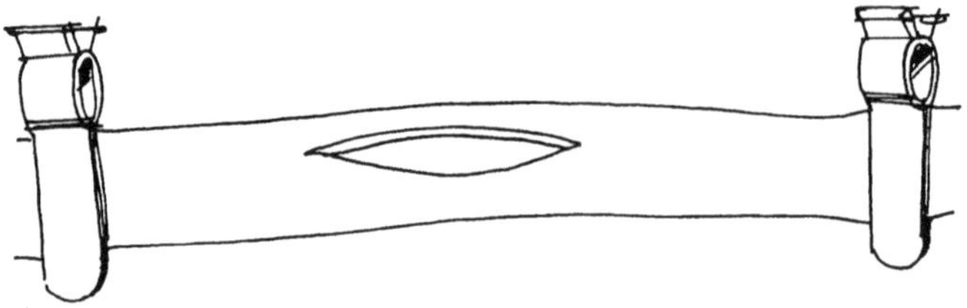

without

or

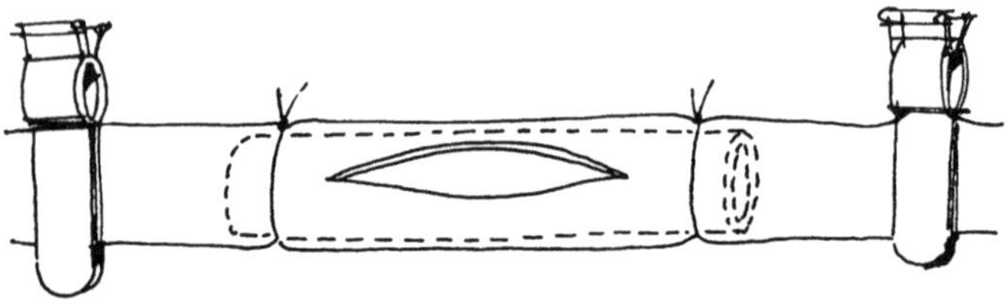

with tube

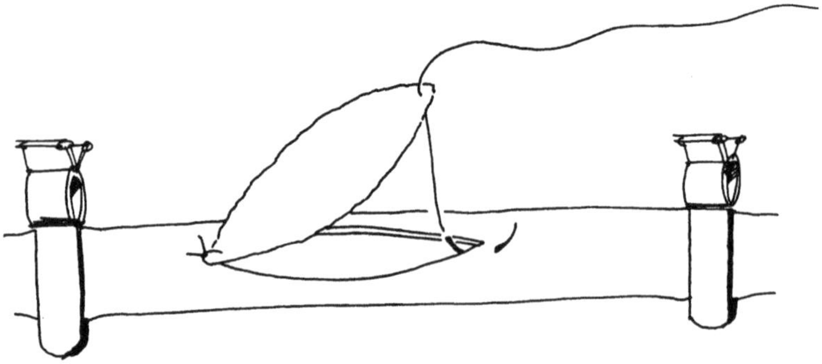

First the two fixation sutures

Then suture of the opposite side:

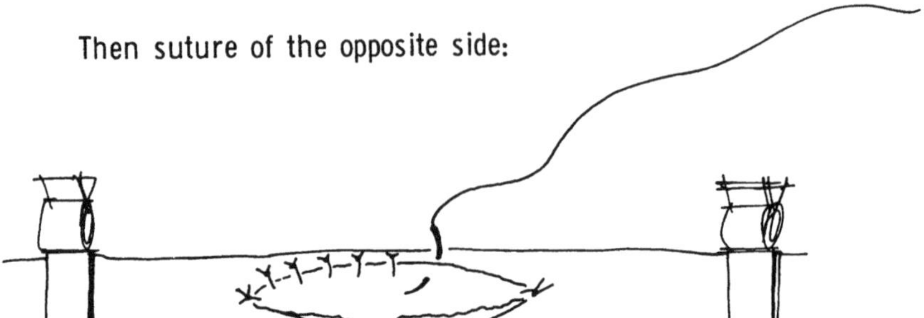

And now the "easy" side:

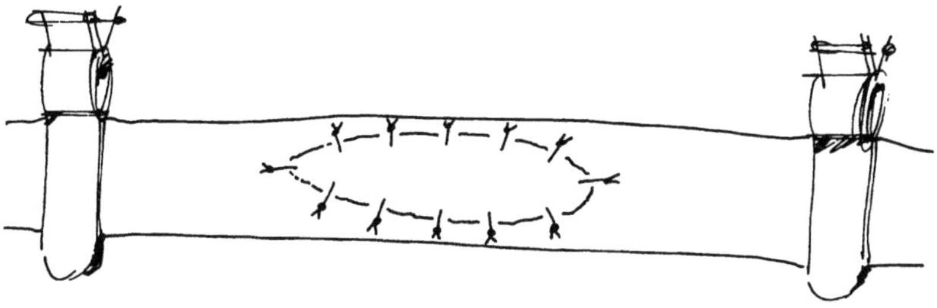

if you use a tube: remove it and flush the clipped vessel as described before.

Variation: Continuous suture.

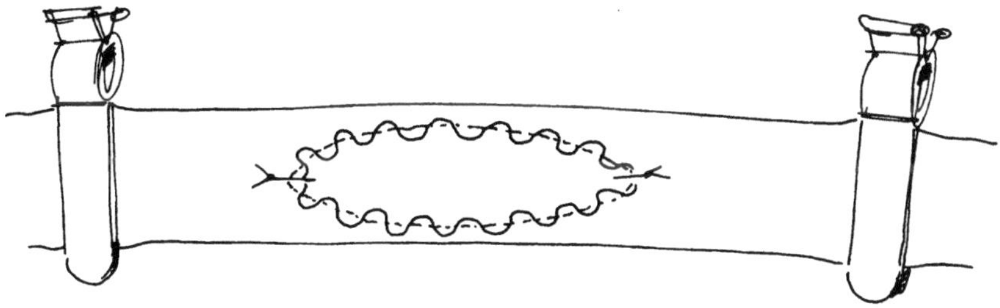

5) End to side anastomosis with a section of a vein.

A) Preparation of the vein:

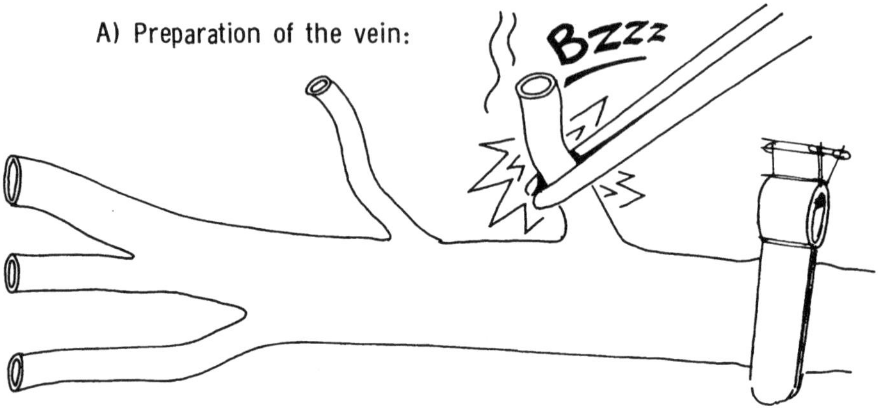

Jugular vein

Clip the jugular vein as proximal as possible.
Occlude all the branches by tying or bipolar coagulation and cut them off.

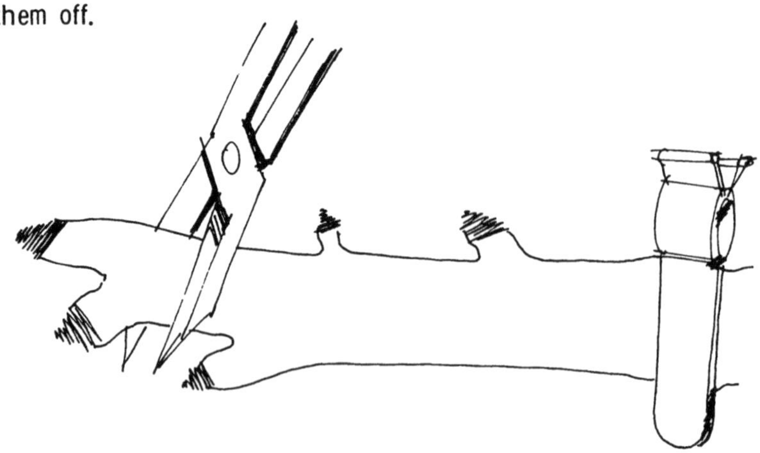

Now cut the vein and flush the blood out with heparin solution.

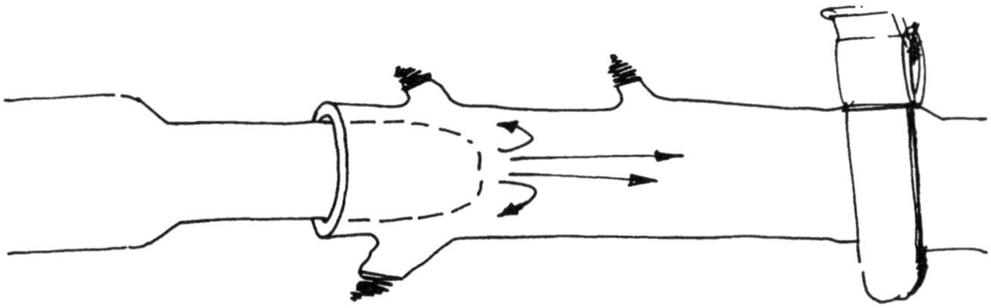

Then insert a tube and fix it slightly:

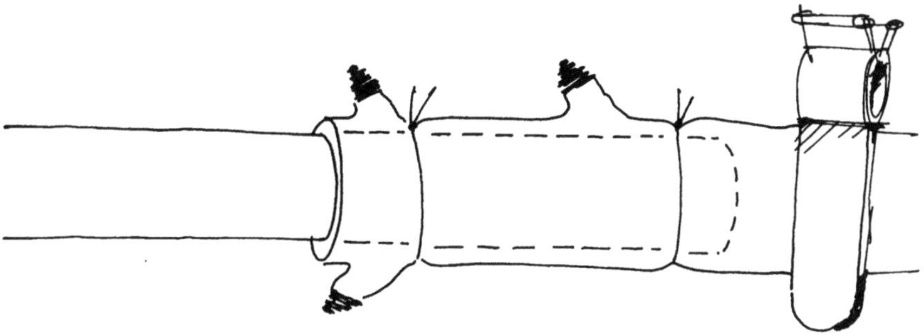

Now cut off the vein:

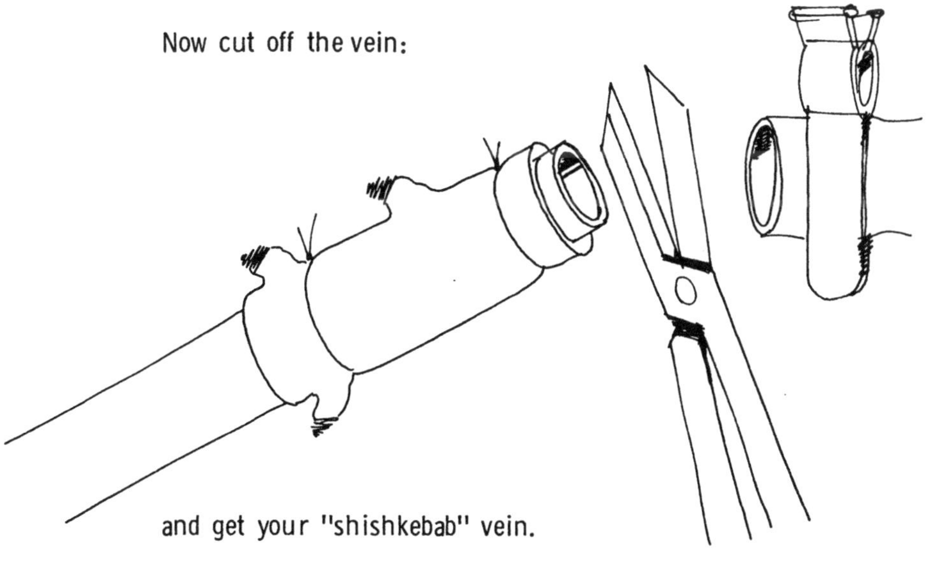

and get your "shishkebab" vein.

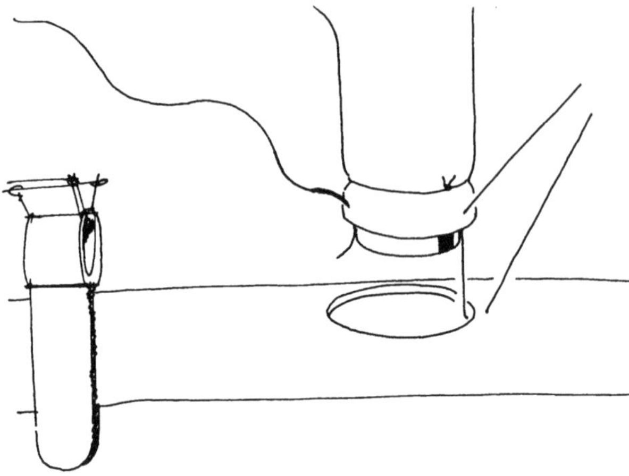

Approximation of the "shishkebab" vein.

Prepared carotid artery with oval excision with or without tube.

Set again the first two fixation sutures.

Then suture the circumference, turning the "shishkebab" vein in suitable position:

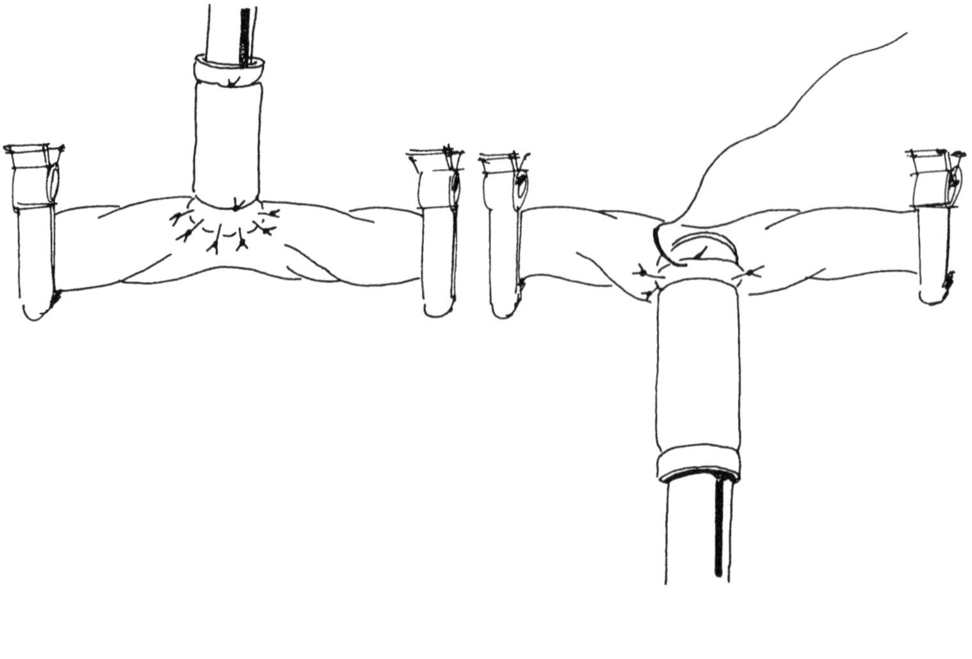

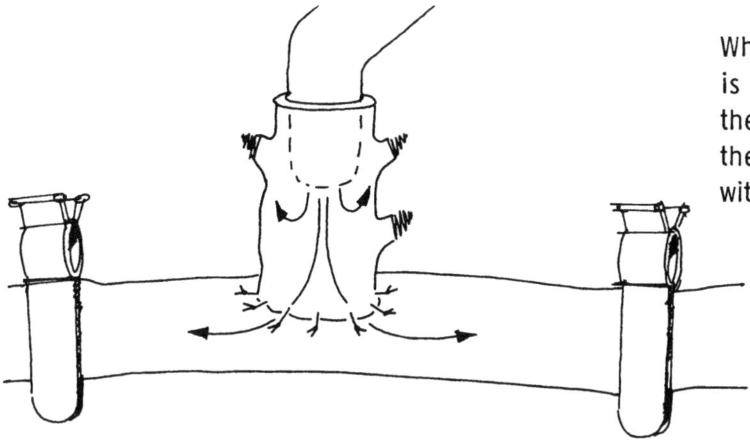

When the anastomosis is finished, remove the tube and flush the whole system with heparin

Then occlude the vein by tying or coagulation:

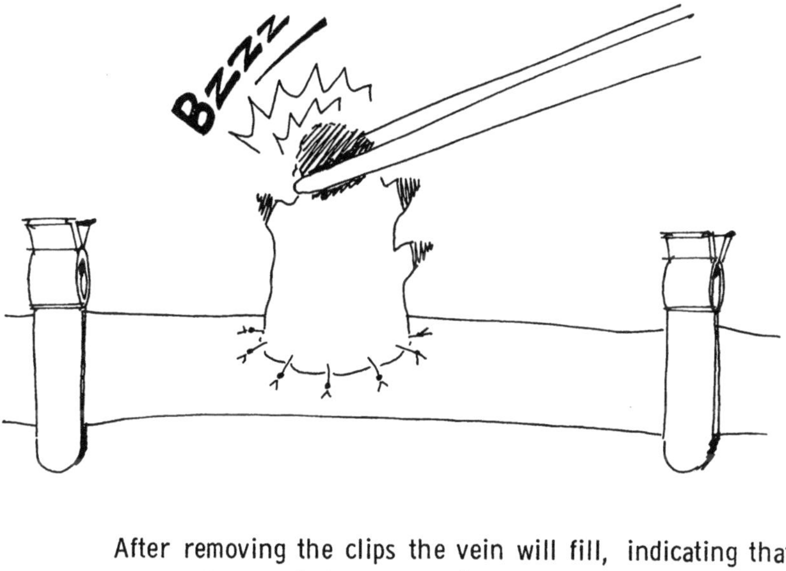

After removing the clips the vein will fill, indicating that you made a perfect anastomosis.

In addition you get one of several "aneurysms" which you may use for later exercise (clipping, bipolar shrinking).

Variation:

End to End Anastomosis with interposition of a vein

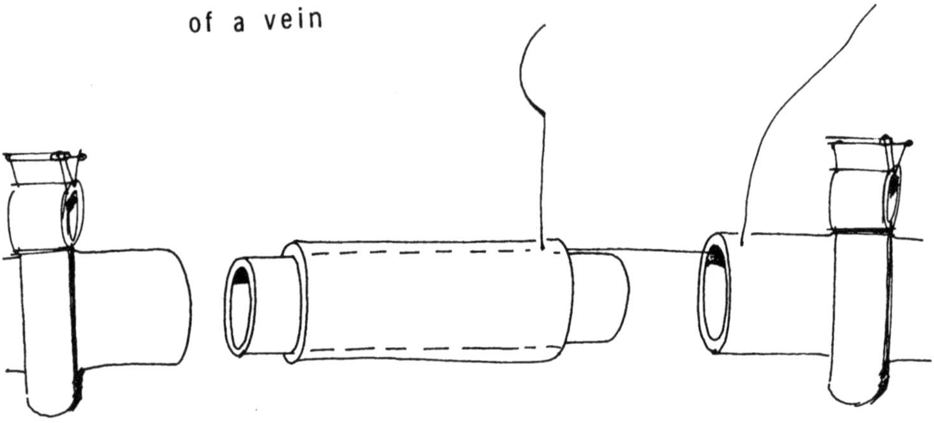

6) Arterio - Venous
End to Side Anastomosis.

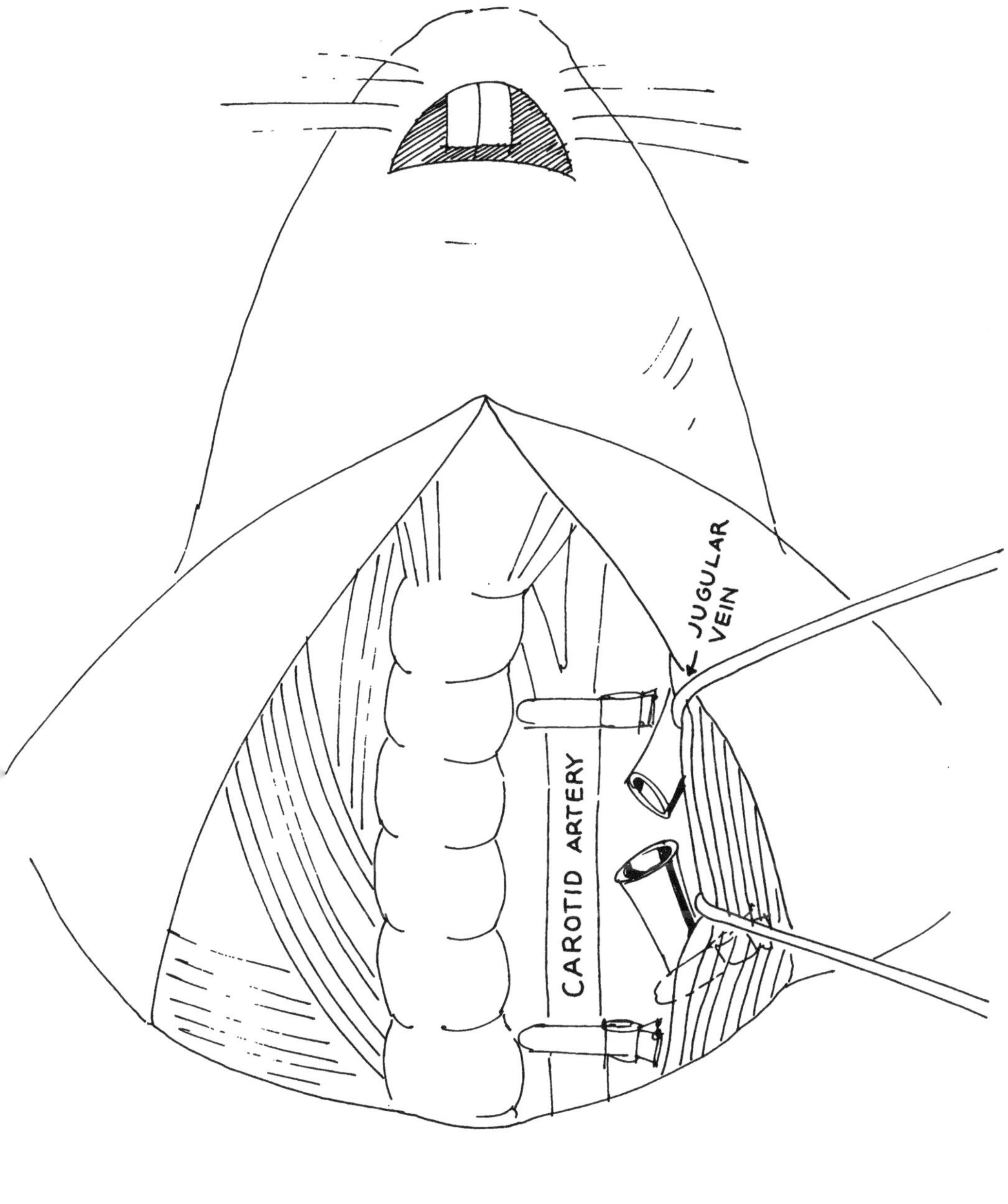

First prepare Jugular Vein:
Clip it as proximal as possible.
Occlude all branches.
Cut the vein off as distal as possible.
Flush the clipped stump with heparin .

Second prepare the Carotid Artery:
Clip it as proximal and distal as possible.
Place the rubber sheet under the artery.
Make the oval excision and flush the blood out with heparin .

Now approximate the vein lumen to the artery:

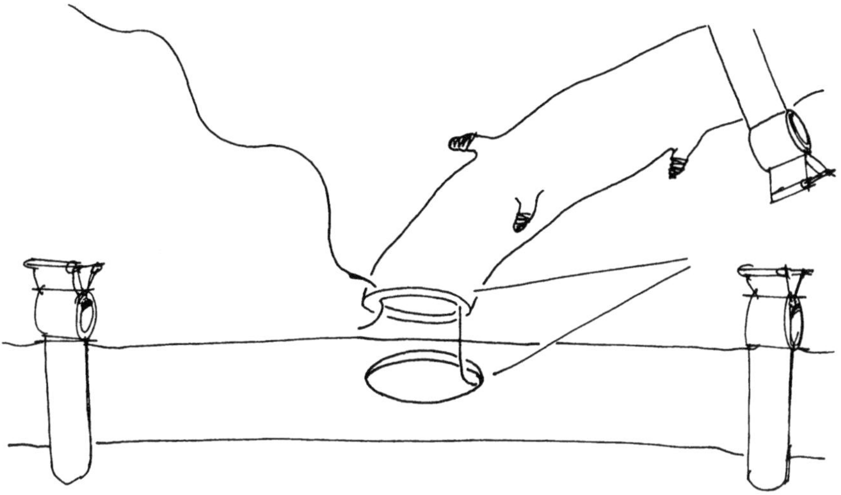

You may use a flexible T-tube:

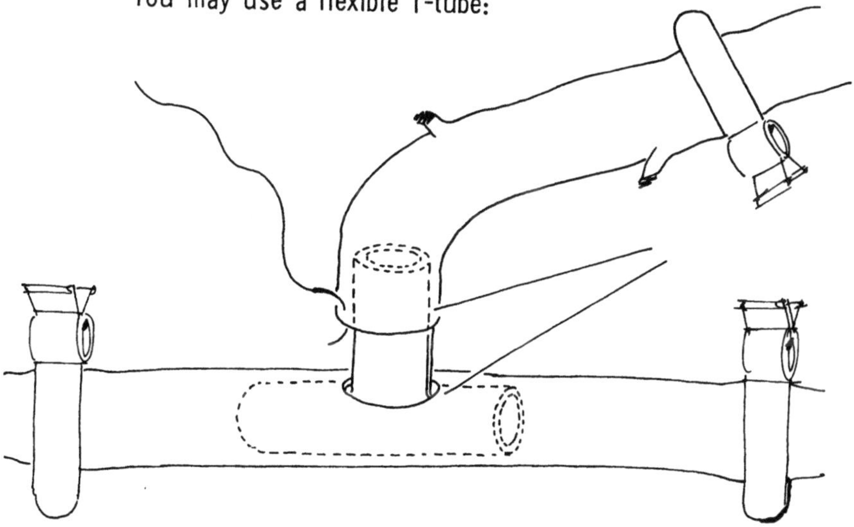

<u>B U T</u> (in our experience) it has

disadvantages:
you may damage the intima inserting and removing the tube.
You may damage your suture when you remove the tube.

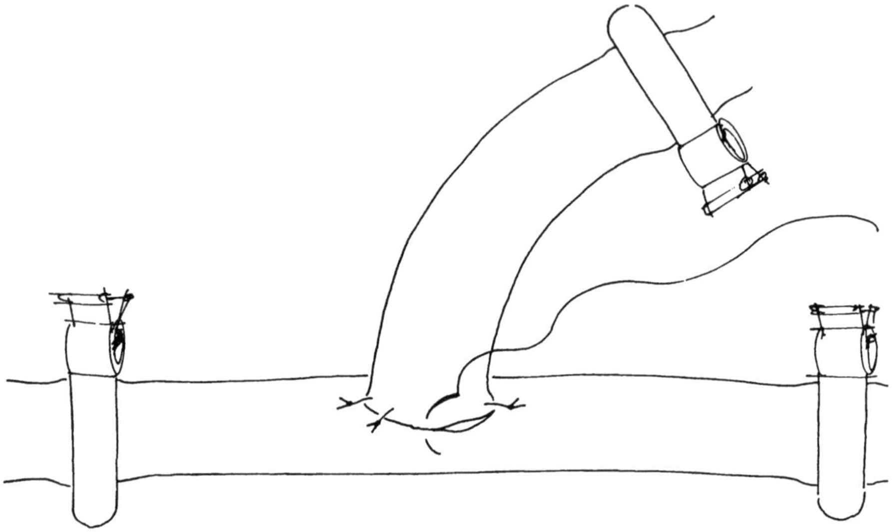

Usually you perform first the suture on the "easy" upside.

Sometimes you will find some difficulties to suture the opposite side.

At that moment you will realize, that it is important, to have a long venous vessel!

If the stump of the vein is long enough you can turn it over:

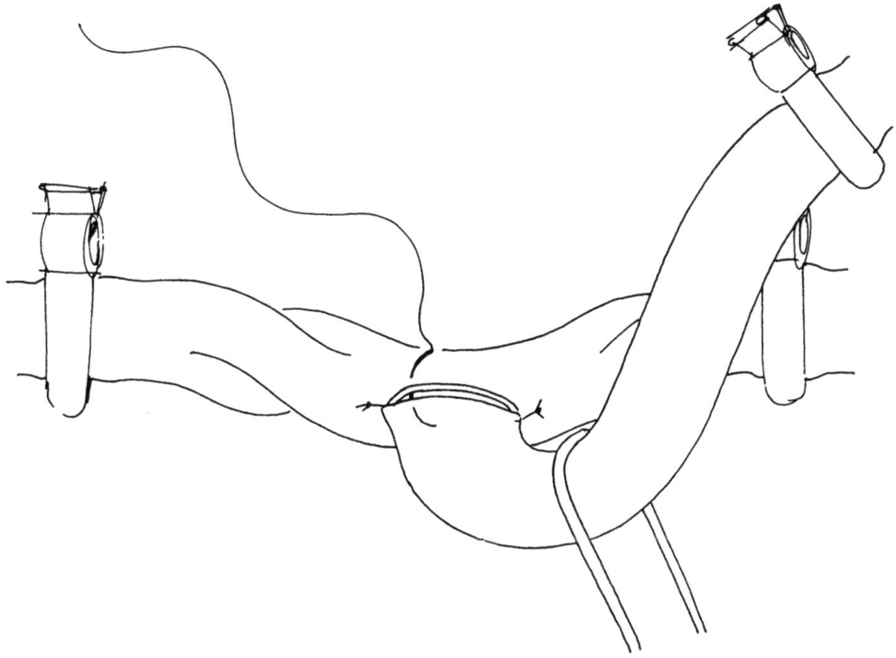

Before setting and tying the last two sutures flush with heparin solution.

When your anastomosis is finished, remove first the venous clip. Then the distal clip from the artery and last the proximal arterial clip.

You may get some bleeding from the anastomosis, but slight compression for 3-4 minutes will stop it, until the "welcomed" external thrombus has developed .

Heavy compression usually leads to the internal thrombus and to occlusion of the anastomosis.

Further suggestions:

1.) Avoid the compression of the trachea.

2.) You may close the wound and let the animal survive the experiment. After 2-3 weeks expose your anastomosis again.
If you have X-Ray facilities, check your anastomosis by angiography.
If you produced an aneurysm you may train the clipping, dissection and coagulation of the sac.
You may excise the anastomosis. Check the patency, open the carotid (not at the suture line) and look at what you have done from the "inside".

Peripheral nerves

RABBIT

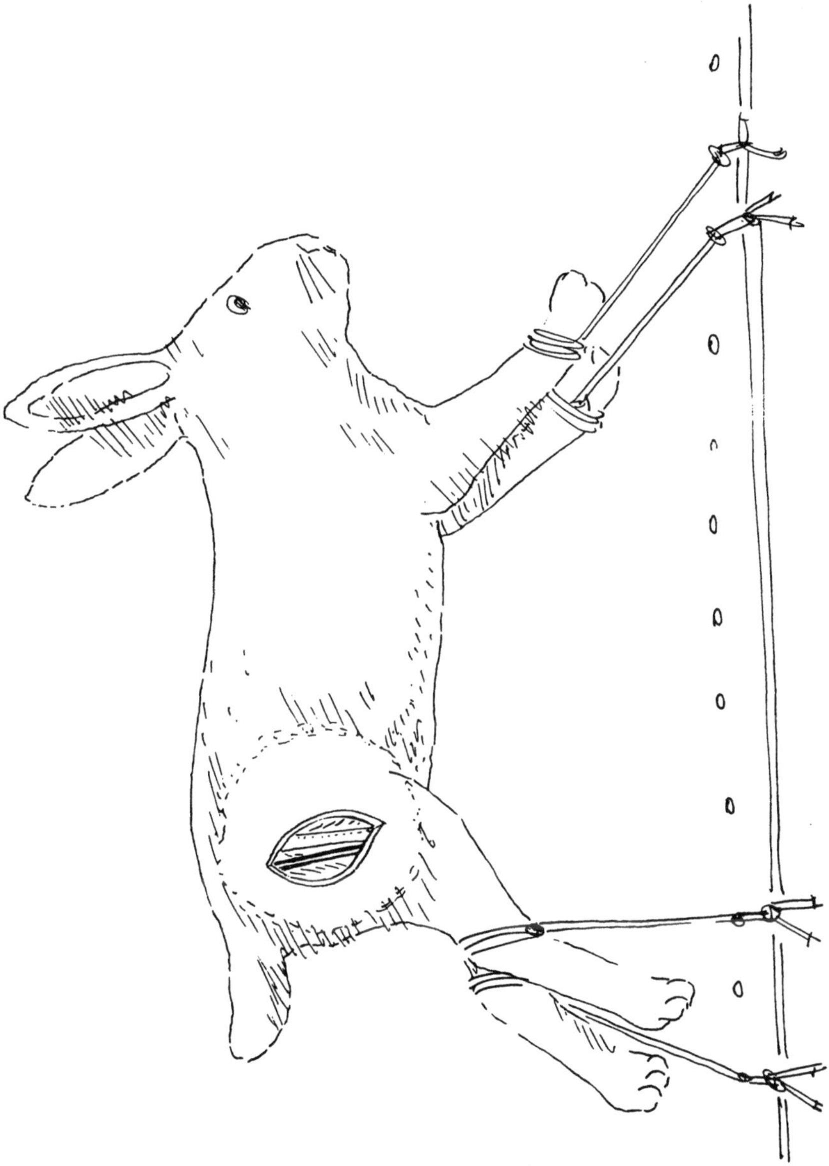

Exposure of the sciatic nerve :

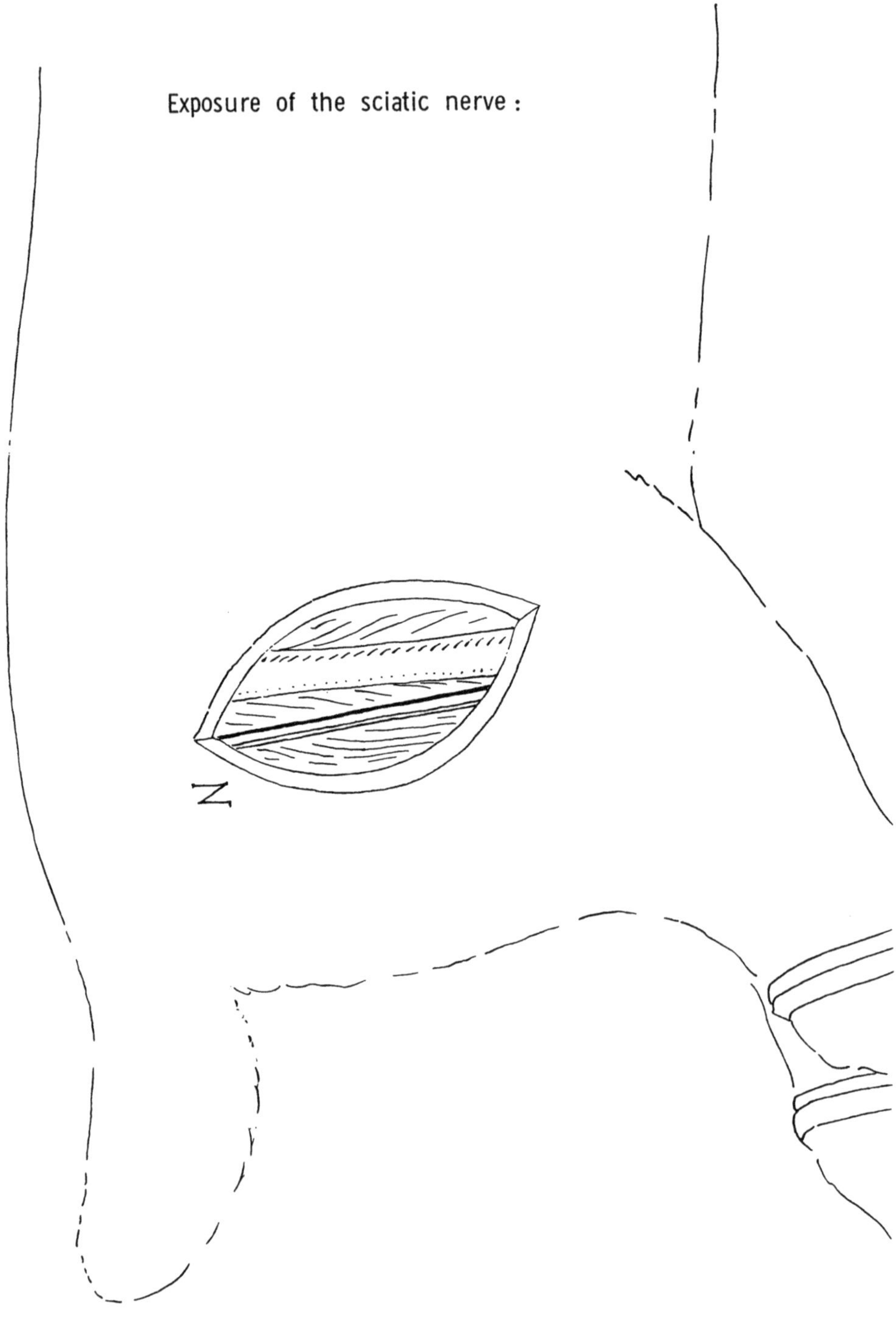

Preparation of the sciatic nerve:

remove surrounding connective tissue and vessels.

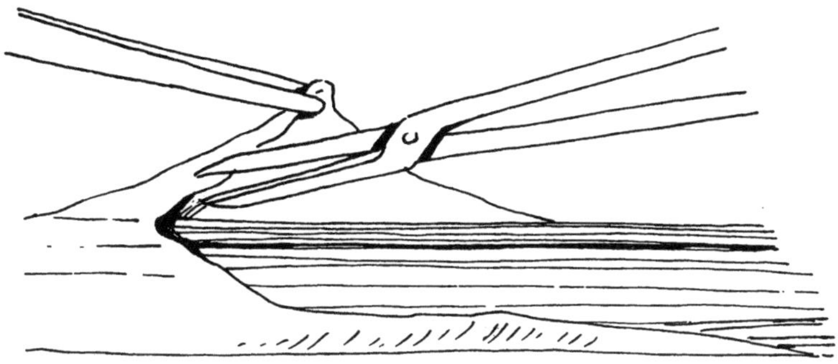

Cut off the nerve:

sometimes it is useful to cut off only the major part, because the intact minor part helps avoid the stumps from retracting too far.

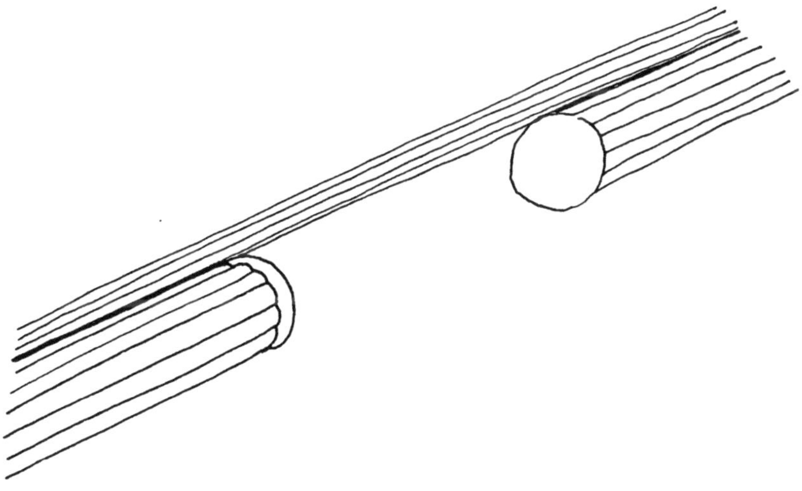

Shortly after cutting, the axoplasma will protrude:

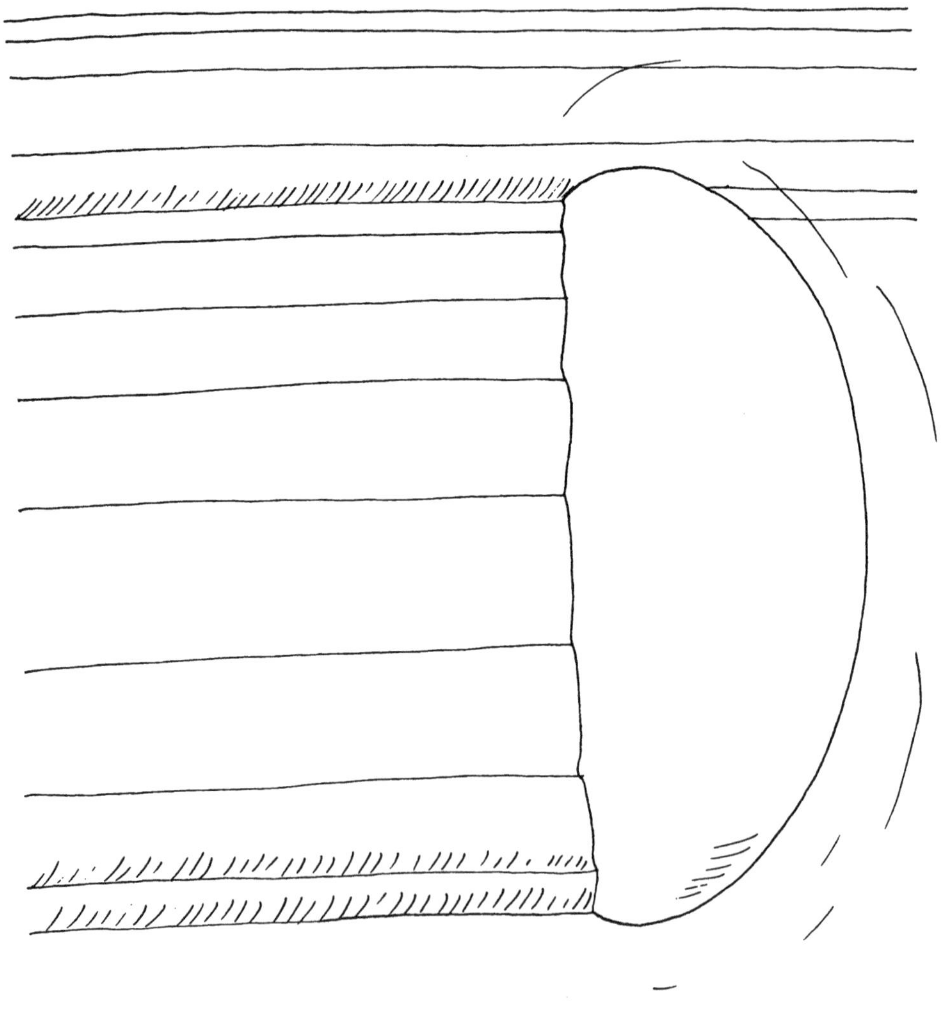

IMPORTANT:

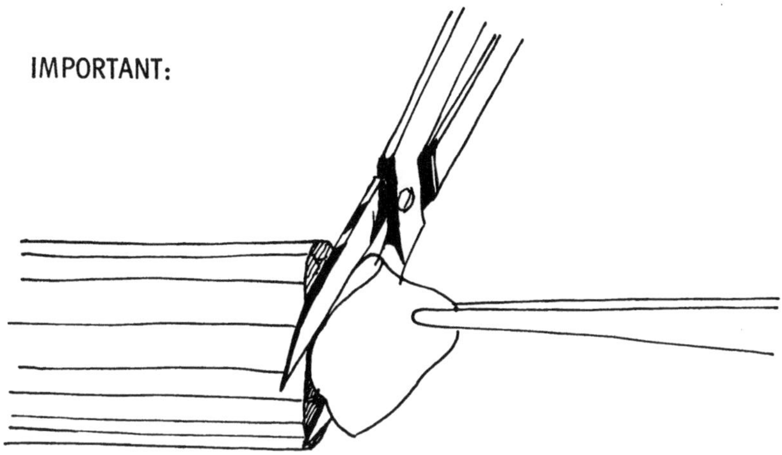

Cut back the protruding axoplasma until the surface of the stumps appears plain and smooth:

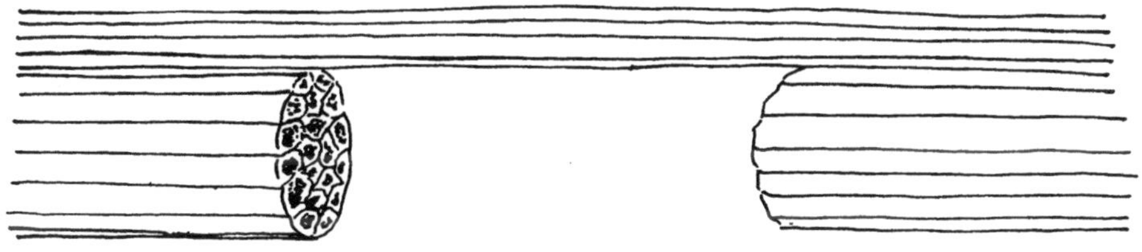

Then set the first two sutures:

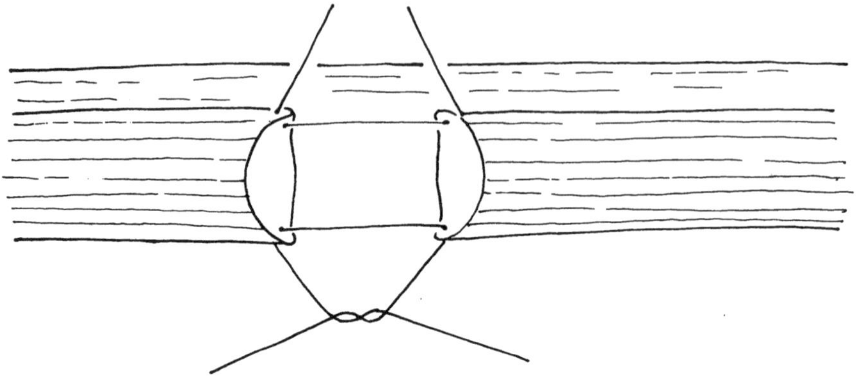

You will sometimes find your skill challenged by the first two sutures because of the tension of the distracted stumps! Going on, you may use the same technique as in end-to-end anastomosis of a vessel: do not cut the thread of the two initial fixation stiches, so that the nerve may later be rotated.

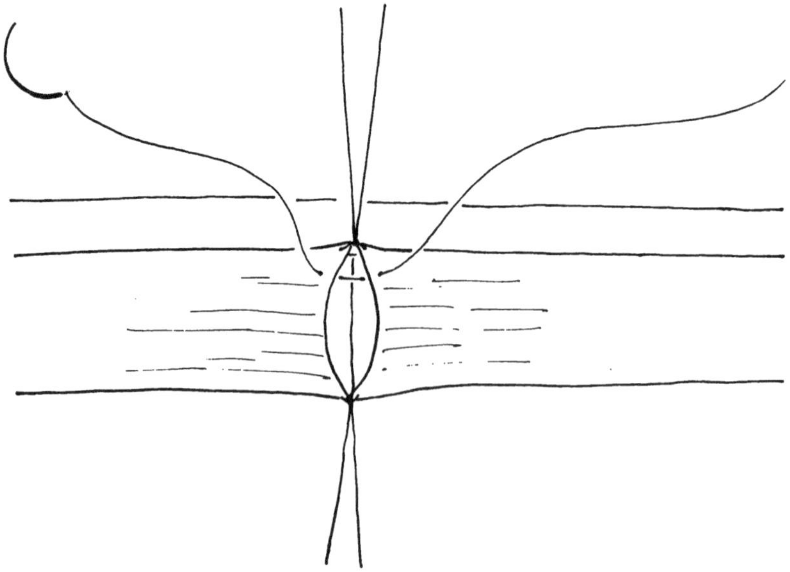

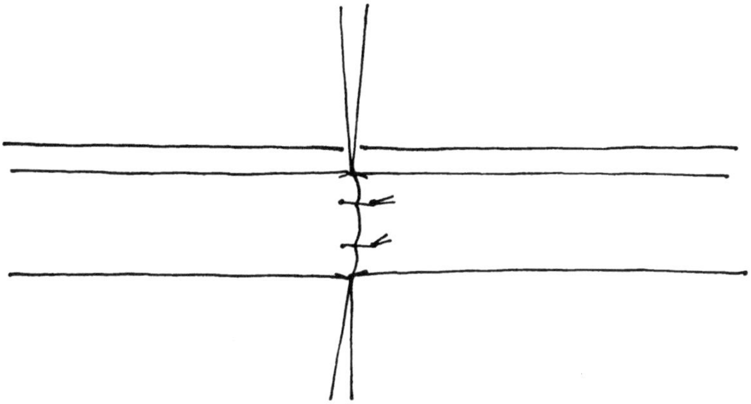

Turn around to suture the opposite side. Usually in anastomosing a nerve, not as many stiches are needed as in anastomosing a vessel.

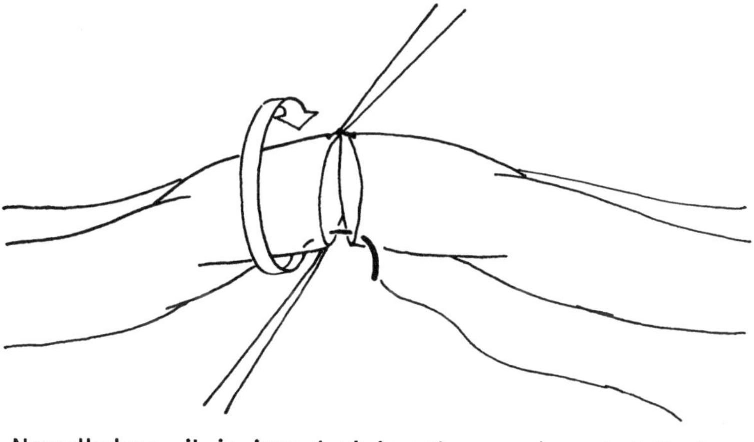

Nevertheless, it is important to get a precise adaptation!

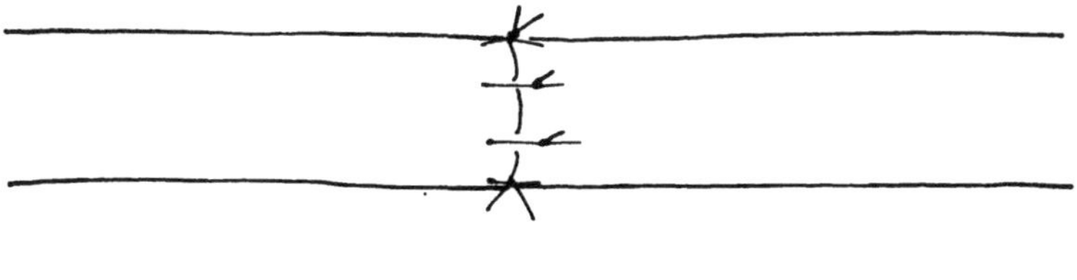

Interposition

First cut out a suitable piece of sciatic nerve, app. lo - 15 mm long.

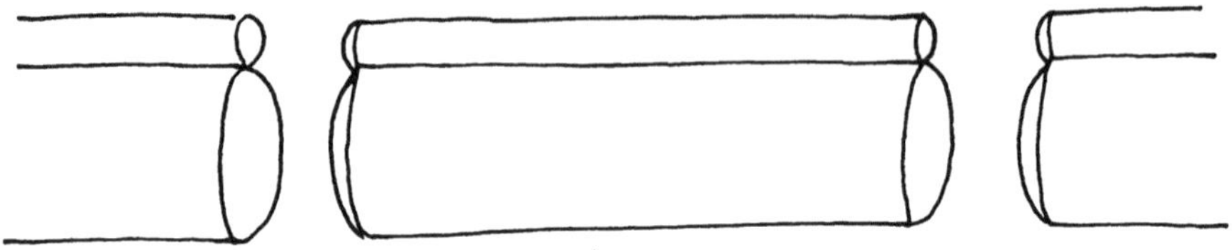

Put the excised piece into saline and prepare the sciatic nerve of the contralateral extremity. This time you may cut both portions of the sciatic nerve.

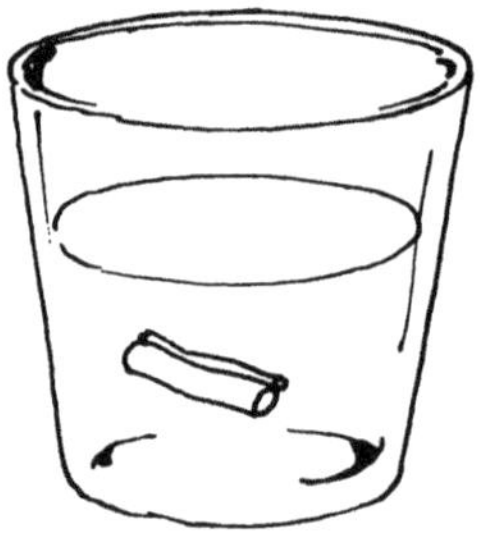

Cut back the axoplasma of the nerve as well as that of the transplant.

Then fit in the transplant between the retracted stumps:

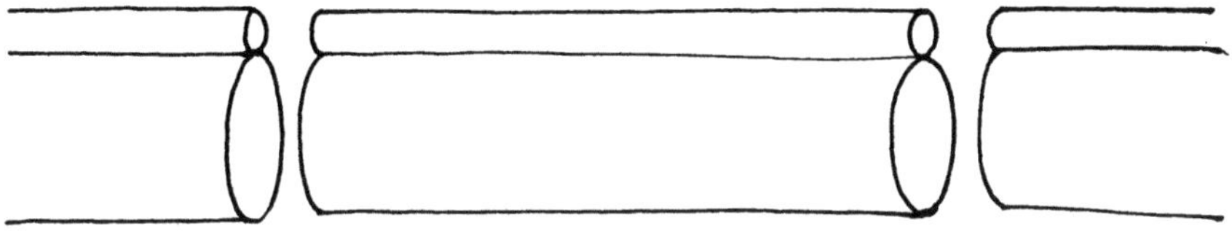

You will find performing the suture a little easier, because this time you won't have any tension (On the other hand, sometimes you will have a sort of "fight" with the very mobile transplant).

Variation:

Interposition of two or three minor portions:

Cut two or three pieces of equal length out of the minor portion of the sciatic nerve:

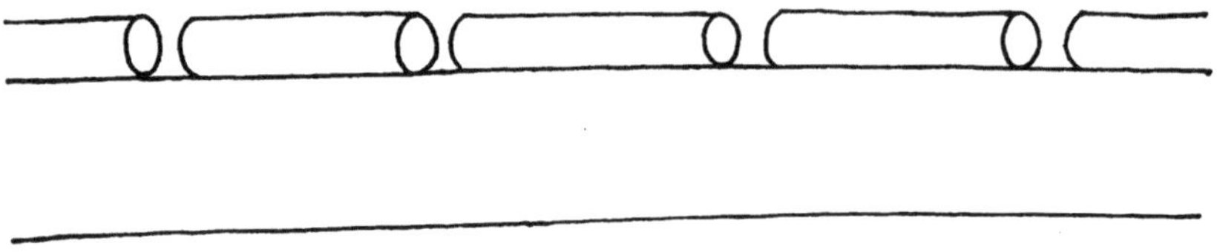

Fit them into the gap between the stumps of the major portion like this....

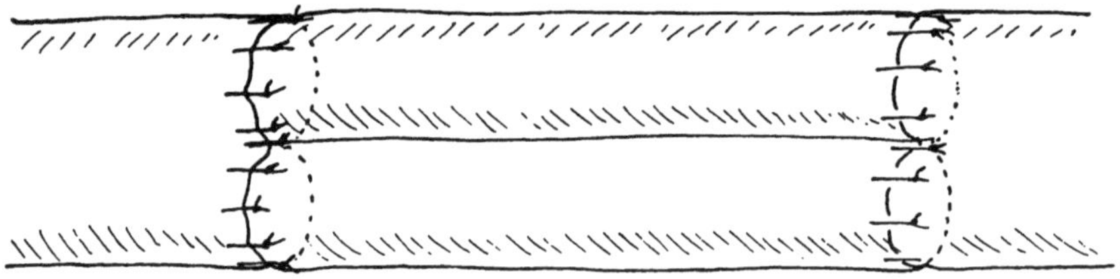

or like this:

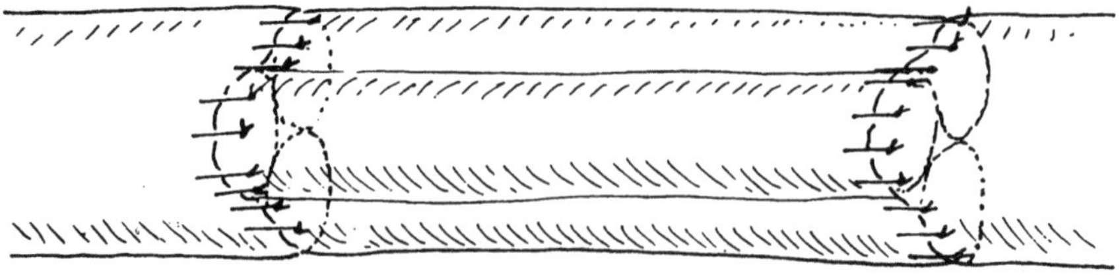

and perform suture.

In our opinion, the animal should be killed after you have finished your operation, because there is no quality of life for a rabbit surviving with paralysed hind limbs.

Bei Fragen zur Produktsicherheit wenden Sie sich bitte an:
If you have any questions regarding product safety,
please contact:

Walter de Gruyter GmbH
Genthiner Straße 13
10785 Berlin
productsafety@degruyterbrill.com